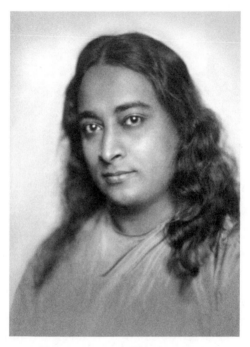

PARAMAHANSA YOGANANDA
(1893–1952)

PARAMAHANSA YOGANANDA

THE
LAW OF SUCCESS

Using the Power

of Spirit to Create

Health, Prosperity,

and Happiness

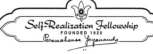

Self-Realization Fellowship
FOUNDED 1920
Paramahansa Yogananda

ABOUT THIS BOOK: *The Law of Success* was first published as a booklet in 1944 by Self-Realization Fellowship, and has been continuously in print since then. It has been translated into five languages: French, German, Italian, Portuguese, and Spanish.

Authorized by the International Publications Council of
SELF-REALIZATION FELLOWSHIP
3880 San Rafael Avenue
Los Angeles, California 90065-3298

The Self-Realization Fellowship name and emblem (shown above) appear on all SRF books, recordings, and other publications, assuring the reader that a work originates with the society established by Paramahansa Yogananda and faithfully conveys his teachings.

Seventh edition, 1980. This printing, 2006.

ISBN-13: 978-0-87612-150-4
ISBN-10: 0-87612-150-4
Printed in the United States of America

1450-J472

He is the wisest who seeks God. He is the most successful who has found God.
　　　　　— *Paramahansa Yogananda*

THE NOBLE NEW

Sing songs that none have sung,
Think thoughts that ne'er in brain have
    rung,
Walk in paths that none have trod,
Weep tears as none have shed for God,
Give peace to all to whom none other
    gave,
Claim him your own who's everywhere
    disclaimed.
Love all with love that none have felt, and
    brave
The battle of life with strength unchained.

My Divine Birthright

The Lord created me in His image. I will seek Him first, and make sure of my actual contact with Him; then, if it be His will, may all things—wisdom, abundance, health—be added as part of my divine birthright.

I want success without measure, not from earthly sources but from God's all-possessing, all-powerful, all-bountiful hands.

THE
LAW OF SUCCESS

——

Is there a power that can reveal hidden veins of riches and uncover treasures of which we never dreamed? Is there a force that we can call upon to give health, happiness, and spiritual enlightenment? The saints and sages of India teach that there is such a power. They have demonstrated the efficacy of truth principles that will work for you, too, if you give them a fair trial.

Your success in life does not altogether depend on ability and training; it also depends on your determination to grasp opportunities that are presented to you. Opportunities in life come by creation, not by chance. You yourself, either now or in the past (including the past of former lives), have created all opportunities that arise in your path. Since you have earned them, use them to the best advantage.

If you use all available outward means, as well as your natural abilities, to overcome every obstacle in your path, you will thus develop the powers that God gave you—unlimited powers that flow from the innermost forces of your being. You possess the power of thought and the power of will. Utilize to the uttermost these divine gifts!

THE POWER OF THOUGHT

You demonstrate success or failure according to your habitual trend of thought. In you which is the stronger—success thoughts or failure thoughts? If your mind is ordinarily in a negative state, an occasional positive thought is not sufficient to attract success. But if you think rightly, you will find your goal even though you seem to be enveloped in darkness.

You alone are responsible for yourself. No one else may answer for your deeds when the final reckoning comes. Your work in the world—in the sphere where your karma, your own past activity, has placed you—can be performed only by one person—yourself. And your work can be called a "success" only when in some way it serves your fellowman.

Don't mentally review any problem constantly. Let it rest at times and it may work itself out; but see that *you* do not rest so long that your discrimination is lost. Rather, use these rest periods to go deep within the calm region of your inner Self. Attuned with your soul, you will be able to think correctly regarding everything you do; and if your thoughts or actions have gone astray they can be realigned. This power of divine attunement can be achieved by practice and effort.

WILL IS THE DYNAMO

Along with positive thinking, you should use will power and continuous activity in order to be successful. Every outward manifestation is the result of will, but this power is not always used consciously. There is mechanical will as well as conscious will. The dynamo of all your powers is volition, or will power. Without volition you cannot walk, talk, work, think, or feel. Therefore will power is the spring of all your actions. (In order not to use this energy, you would have to be completely inactive both physically and mentally. Even when you move your hand, you are using will power. It is impossible to live without using this force.)

Mechanical will is an unthinking use of

7

will power. Conscious will is a vital force accompanying determination and effort, a dynamo that should be wisely directed. As you train yourself to use conscious, not mechanical, will, you should also be sure that your will power is being used constructively, not for harmful purposes nor for useless acquisitions.

To create dynamic will power, determine to do some of the things in life that you thought you could not do. Attempt simple tasks first. As your confidence strengthens and your will becomes more dynamic, you can aim for more difficult accomplishments. Be certain that you have made a good selection, then refuse to submit to failure. Devote your entire will power to mastering one thing at a time; do not scatter your energies, nor leave something half done to begin a new venture.

YOU CAN CONTROL DESTINY

Mind is the creator of everything. You should therefore guide it to create only good. If you cling to a certain thought with dynamic will power, it finally assumes a tangible outward form. When you are able to employ your will always for constructive purposes, you become the *controller of your destiny.*

I have just mentioned three important ways to make your will dynamic: (1) choose a simple task or an accomplishment that you have never mastered and determine to succeed with it; (2) be sure you have chosen something constructive and feasible, then refuse to consider failure; (3) concentrate on a single purpose, using all abilities and opportunities to forward it.

But you should always be sure, within the calm region of your inner Self, that what you want is right for you to have, and in accord with God's purposes. You can then use all the force of your will to accomplish your object; keeping your mind, however, centered on the thought of God—the Source of all power and all accomplishment.

FEAR EXHAUSTS LIFE ENERGY

The human brain is a storehouse of life energy. This energy is constantly employed in muscular movements; in the working of the heart, lungs, and diaphragm; in cellular metabolism and chemicalization of blood; and in carrying on the work of the telephonic sensory motor system (the nerves). Besides this, a tremendous amount of life energy is required in all processes of thought, emotion, and will.

Fear exhausts life energy; it is one of the greatest enemies of dynamic will power. Fear causes the life force that ordinarily flows steadily through the nerves to be squeezed out, and the nerves themselves to become as though paralyzed; the vitality of the whole body is lowered. Fear doesn't help you to get away from the object of fear; it only weakens your will power. Fear causes the brain to send an

are crowned with success. A little story will make this point clear.

A and B were fighting. After a long time A said to himself: "I cannot go on any longer." But B thought: "Just one more punch," and he gave it, and down went A. You must be like that; give a last punch. Use the unconquerable power of will to overcome all difficulties in life.

New efforts after failure bring true growth. But they must be well planned and charged with increasing intensity of attention and with dynamic will power.

Suppose you *have* failed so far. It would be foolish to give up the struggle, accepting failure as the decree of "fate." It is better to die struggling than to abandon your efforts while there is still a possibility of accomplishing something more; for even when death comes, your struggles must soon be renewed in another life. Success or failure is the just result of what you have done in the past, *plus* what you do now. So you should stimulate all the success thoughts of past lives until they are revitalized and able to overrule the influence of all failure tendencies in the present life.

The successful person may have had more serious difficulties to contend with than one who has failed, but the former trains himself to reject the thought of failure at all times. You should transfer your attention from failure to success, from worry to calmness, from mental wanderings to concentration, from restlessness to peace, and from peace to the divine bliss within. When you attain this state of Self-realization the purpose of your life will have been gloriously fulfilled.

The Need for Self-Analysis

Another secret of progress is self-analysis. Introspection is a mirror in which to see recesses of your mind that otherwise would remain hidden from you. Diagnose your failures and sort out your good and bad tendencies. Analyze what you are, what you wish to become, and what shortcomings are impeding you. Decide the nature of your true task — your mission in life. Endeavor to make yourself what you should be and what you want to be. As you keep your mind on God and attune your-self to His will, you will progress more and more surely in your path.

Your ultimate purpose is to find your way back to God, but you also have a task to perform in the outer world. Will power, combined with initiative, will help you to recognize and fulfill that task.

THE CREATIVE POWER OF INITIATIVE

What is initiative? It is a creative faculty within you, a spark of the Infinite Creator. It may give you the power to create some-thing no one else has ever created. It urges you to do things in new ways. The accom-plishments of a person of initiative may be as spectacular as a shooting star. Apparently creating something from nothing, he demonstrates that the seemingly impossible may become possible by one's employment of the great inventive power of the Spirit.

Initiative enables you to stand on your own feet, free and independent. It is one of the attributes of success.

SEE THE IMAGE OF GOD IN ALL MEN

Many people excuse their own faults but judge other persons harshly. We should reverse this attitude by excusing others' shortcomings and by harshly examining our own.

Sometimes it is necessary to analyze other people; in that case the important thing to remember is to keep the mind unprejudiced. An unbiased mind is like a clear mirror, held steady, not oscillating with hasty judgments. Any person reflected within that mirror will present an undistorted image.

Learn to see God in all persons, of whatever race or creed. You will know what divine love is when you begin to feel your oneness with every human being, not before. In mutual service we forget the little self, and glimpse the one measureless Self, the Spirit that unifies all men.

HABITS OF THOUGHT
CONTROL ONE'S LIFE

—

Success is hastened or delayed by one's habits.

It is not your passing inspirations or brilliant ideas so much as your everyday mental habits that control your life. Habits of thought are mental magnets that draw to you certain things, people, and conditions. Good habits of thought enable you to attract benefits and opportunities. Bad habits of thought attract you to materially minded persons and to unfavorable environments.

Weaken a bad habit by avoiding everything that occasioned it or stimulated it, *without concentrating upon it in your zeal to avoid it.* Then divert your mind to some good habit and steadily cultivate it until it becomes a dependable part of you.

There are always two forces warring against each other within us. One force tells us to do the things we should not do; and the other urges us to do the things we should do, the things that seem difficult. One voice is that of evil, and the other is that of good, or God.

Through difficult daily lessons you will sometime see clearly that bad habits nourish the tree of unending material desires, while good habits nourish the tree of spiritual aspirations. More and more you should concentrate your efforts on successfully maturing the spiritual tree, that you may someday gather the ripe fruit of Self-realization.

If you are able to free yourself from all kinds of bad habits, and if you are able to do good because you want to do good and not merely because evil brings sorrow, then you are truly progressing in Spirit.

It is only when you discard your bad habits that you are really a free man. Until you are a true master, able to command yourself to do the things that you should do but may not want to do, you are not a free soul. *In that power of self-control lies the seed of eternal freedom.*

I have now mentioned several important attributes of success — positive thoughts, dynamic will, self-analysis, initiative, and self-control. Many popular books stress one or more of these, but fail to give credit to the Divine Power behind them. *Attunement with the Divine Will is the most important factor in attracting success.*

Divine Will is the power that moves the cosmos and everything in it. It was God's will that hurled the stars into space. It is His will that holds the planets in their orbits and that directs the cycles of birth, growth, and decay in all forms of life.

POWER OF DIVINE WILL

Divine Will has no boundaries; it works through laws known and unknown, natural and seemingly miraculous. It can change the course of destiny, wake the dead, cast mountains into the sea, and create new solar systems.

Man, as an image of God, possesses within him that all-accomplishing power of will. To discover through right meditation* how to be in harmony with the Divine Will is man's highest obligation.

When guided by error, human will misleads us; but when guided by wisdom, human will is attuned to the Divine Will. God's plan for us often becomes obscured by the conflicts of human life and so we lose the inner guidance that would save us

---

* Meditation is that special form of concentration in which the attention has been liberated, by scientific yoga techniques, from the restlessness of the body-conscious state, and is focused one-pointedly on God. The *Self-Realization Fellowship Lessons* give detailed instruction in this science of meditation. *(Publisher's Note)*

from chasms of misery.

Jesus said: "Thy will be done." When man attunes his will with God's will, which is guided by wisdom, he is using Divine Will. Through the use of right techniques of meditation, developed anciently by India's sages, all men may achieve perfect harmony with the will of the Heavenly Father.

FROM THE OCEAN OF ABUNDANCE

Just as all power lies in His will, so all spiritual and material gifts flow from His boundless abundance. In order to receive His gifts you must eradicate from your mind all thoughts of limitation and poverty. Universal Mind is perfect and knows no lack; to reach that never-failing supply you must maintain a consciousness of abundance. Even when you do not know where the next dollar is coming from, you should refuse to be apprehensive. When you do your part and rely on God to do His, you will find that mysterious forces come to your aid and that your constructive wishes soon materialize. This confidence and consciousness of abundance are attained through meditation.

Since God is the source of all mental power, peace, and prosperity, *do not will and act first, but contact God first.* Thus you may harness your will and activity to achieve the highest goals. As you cannot broadcast through a broken microphone, so you cannot send out prayers through a mental microphone that has been disordered by restlessness. By deep calmness you should repair your mind microphone and increase the receptivity of your intuition. Thus you will be able to broadcast to Him effectively and to receive His answers.

THE WAY OF MEDITATION

After you have repaired your mental radio and are calmly attuned to constructive vibrations, how may you use it to reach God? The right method of meditation is the way.

By the power of concentration and meditation you can direct the inexhaustible power of your mind to accomplish what you desire and to guard every door against failure. All successful men and women devote much time to deep concentration. They are able to dive deeply within their minds and to find the pearls of right solutions for the problems that confront them. If you learn how to withdraw your attention from all objects of distraction and to place it upon one object of concentration, you too will know how to attract at will whatever you need.

Before embarking on important undertakings, sit quietly, calm your senses and thoughts, and meditate deeply. You will then be guided by the great creative power of Spirit. After that you should utilize all necessary material means to achieve your goal.

The things you need in life are those

that will help to fulfill your dominant purpose. Things you may *want* but not *need* may lead you aside from that purpose. It is only by making everything serve your main objective that success is attained.

SUCCESS IS MEASURED BY HAPPINESS

Consider whether fulfillment of the goal you have chosen will constitute success. What *is* success? If you possess health and wealth, but have trouble with everybody (including yourself), yours is not a successful life. Existence becomes futile if you cannot find happiness. *When wealth is lost, you have lost a little; when health is lost, you have lost something of more conse-*

*quence; but when peace of mind is lost, you
have lost the highest treasure.*

Success should therefore be measured by
the yardstick of happiness; by your ability
to remain in peaceful harmony with cosmic
laws. Success is not rightly measured by the
worldly standards of wealth, prestige, and
power. None of these bestow happiness
unless they are rightly used. To use them
rightly one must possess wisdom and love
for God and man.

God does not reward or punish you. He
has given you the power to reward or punish yourself by the use or misuse of your
own reason and will power. If you trans-
gress the laws of health, prosperity, and wisdom you must inevitably suffer from sick-
ness, poverty, and ignorance. However, you

should strengthen your mind and refuse to carry the burden of mental and moral weaknesses acquired in past years; burn them in the fires of your present divine resolutions and right activities. By this constructive attitude you will attain freedom.

Happiness depends to some extent upon external conditions, but chiefly upon mental attitudes. In order to be happy one should have good health, a well-balanced mind, a prosperous life, the right work, a thankful heart, and, above all, wisdom or knowledge of God.

A strong determination to be happy will help you. Do not wait for your circumstances to change, thinking falsely that in them lies the trouble. Do not make unhappiness a chronic habit, thereby afflicting yourself and your associates. It is blessed-ness for yourself and others if you are happy. If you possess happiness you possess everything; to be happy is to be in tune with God. That power to be happy comes through meditation.

PUT GOD'S POWER BEHIND YOUR EFFORTS

Release for constructive purposes the power you already have, and more will come. Move on your path with unflinching determination, using all the attributes of success. Tune yourself with the creative power of Spirit. You will be in contact with the Infinite Intelligence that is able to guide you and to solve all problems. Power from the dynamic Source of your being will flow uninterruptedly so that you will be able to perform creatively in any sphere of activity.

You should sit in silence before deciding about any important matter, asking the Father for His blessing. Then behind your power is God's power; behind your mind, His mind; behind your will, His will. When God is working with you, you cannot fail; every faculty you possess will increase in power. When you do your work with the thought of serving God, you receive His blessings.

If your work in life is humble, do not apologize for it. Be proud because you are fulfilling the duty given you by the Father. He needs you in your particular place; all people cannot play the same role. So long as you work to please God, all cosmic forces will harmoniously assist you.

When you convince God that you want Him above all else, you will be attuned to His will. When you continue to seek Him no matter what obstacles arise to take you away from Him, you are using your human will in its most constructive form. You will thus operate the law of success that was known to the ancient sages and that is understood by all men who have achieved true success. The divine power is yours if you make a determined effort to use it to attain health, happiness, and peace. As you encompass these goals you will travel on the path of Self-realization to your true home in God.

AFFIRMATION

Heavenly Father, I will reason, I will will, I will act; but guide Thou my reason, will, and activity to the right thing that I should do.

ABOUT THE AUTHOR

Paramahansa Yogananda (1893–1952) is widely regarded as one of the preeminent spiritual figures of our time. Born in northern India, he came to the United States in 1920. Over the next three decades he contributed in far-reaching ways to a greater awareness and appreciation in the West of the perennial wisdom of the East— through his writings, extensive lecture tours, and the creation of numerous Self-Realization Fellowship temples and meditation centers. His acclaimed life story, *Autobiography of a Yogi,* as well as his numerous other books and his comprehensive series of lessons for home study, have introduced millions to India's ancient science of meditation and methods of attaining balanced well-being of body, mind, and soul. Under the guidance of one of his earliest and closest disciples, Sri Daya Mata, his spiritual and humanitarian work is carried on today by Self-Realization Fellowship, the international society he founded in 1920 to disseminate his teachings worldwide.

In the Sanctuary of the Soul: A Guide
to Effective Prayer

Living Fearlessly: Bringing Out
Your Inner Soul Strength

Why God Permits Evil and How to Rise Above It

How You Can Talk With God

Metaphysical Meditations

To Be Victorious in Life

Cosmic Chants

*A complete catalog of books and audio/video recordings
—including rare archival recordings of Paramahansa
Yogananda—is available on request or online at
www.yogananda-srf.org*

SELF-REALIZATION FELLOWSHIP LESSONS

The scientific techniques of meditation taught by
Paramahansa Yogananda, including *Kriya Yoga*—as
well as his guidance on all aspects of balanced spiritual living—are presented in the *Self-Realization
Fellowship Lessons*. For further information, please
ask for the free introductory booklet *Undreamed-of
Possibilities*.

SELF-REALIZATION FELLOWSHIP
3880 San Rafael Avenue • Los Angeles, CA 90065-3298
TEL (323) 225-2471 • FAX (323) 225-5088
www.yogananda-srf.org

AIMS AND IDEALS
OF
SELF-REALIZATION FELLOWSHIP

As set forth by Paramahansa Yogananda, Founder
Sri Daya Mata, President

To disseminate among the nations a knowledge of definite scientific techniques for attaining direct personal experience of God.

To teach that the purpose of life is the evolution, through self-effort, of man's limited mortal consciousness into God Consciousness; and to this end to establish Self-Realization Fellowship temples for God-communion throughout the world, and to encourage the establishment of individual temples of God in the homes and in the hearts of men.

To reveal the complete harmony and basic oneness of original Christianity as taught by Jesus Christ and original Yoga as taught by Bhagavan Krishna; and to show that these principles of truth are the common scientific foundation of all true religions.

To point out the one divine highway to which all paths of true religious beliefs eventually lead: the highway of daily, scientific, devotional meditation on God.

To liberate man from his threefold suffering: physical disease, mental inharmonies, and spiritual ignorance.

To encourage "plain living and high thinking"; and to spread a spirit of brotherhood among all peoples by teaching the eternal basis of their unity: kinship with God.

To demonstrate the superiority of mind over body, of soul over mind.

To overcome evil by good, sorrow by joy, cruelty by kindness, ignorance by wisdom.

To unite science and religion through realization of the unity of their underlying principles.

To advocate cultural and spiritual understanding between East and West, and the exchange of their finest distinctive features.

To serve mankind as one's larger Self.